Chocolate

Aversion Therapy

by S. J. Quast

Chocolate **Aversion Therapy**

Are you addicted to chocolate? Sick of the sugar and serotonin ups and downs? Want to kick the habit to lose weight? Tried everything to stop eating it?

Finally, here is a way to help you help yourself quit for good. This Chocolate Aversion Therapy book is designed by a reformed chocaholic to really put you off it. A series of absolutely revolting pictures to turn off that old desire for the unhealthy. Read the instructions carefully, as the method aims to combine several processes to help you free yourself from wanting or needing chocolate ever again.

Published by S J Quast

ISBN: ISBN-13: 978-1537586373

ISBN-10: 1537586378

IMPORTANT:

read the last 3 pages first.

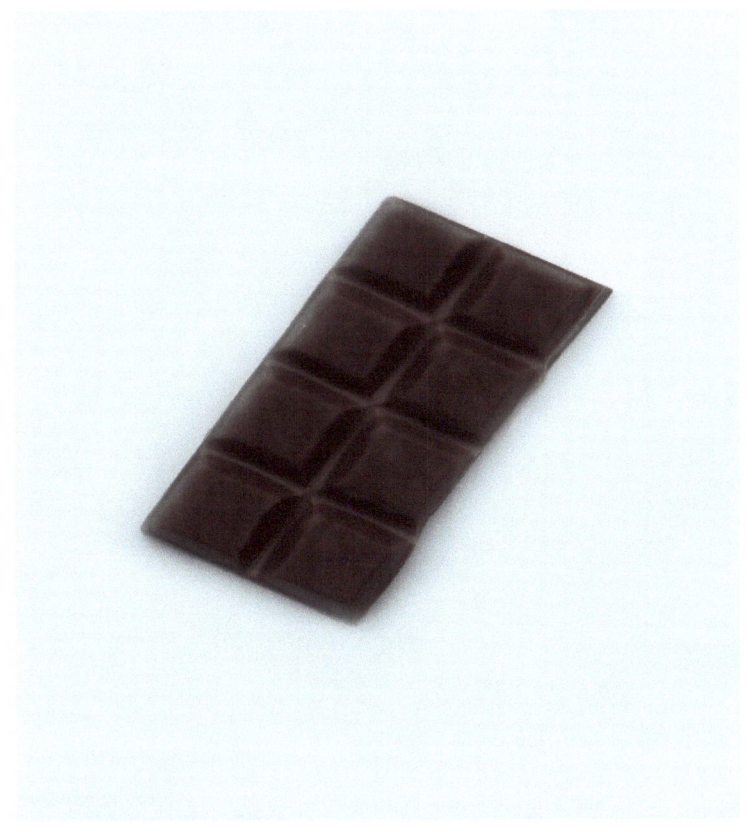

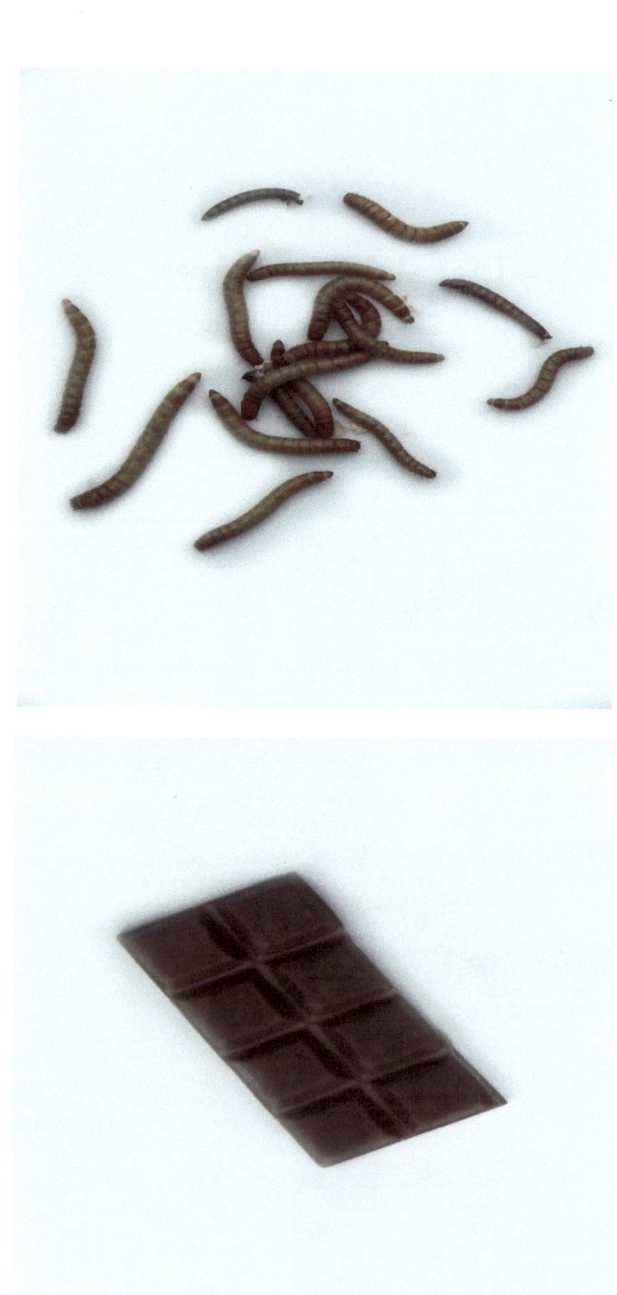

OOEEY! GOOEY!
    Chocolate with mealy worms!

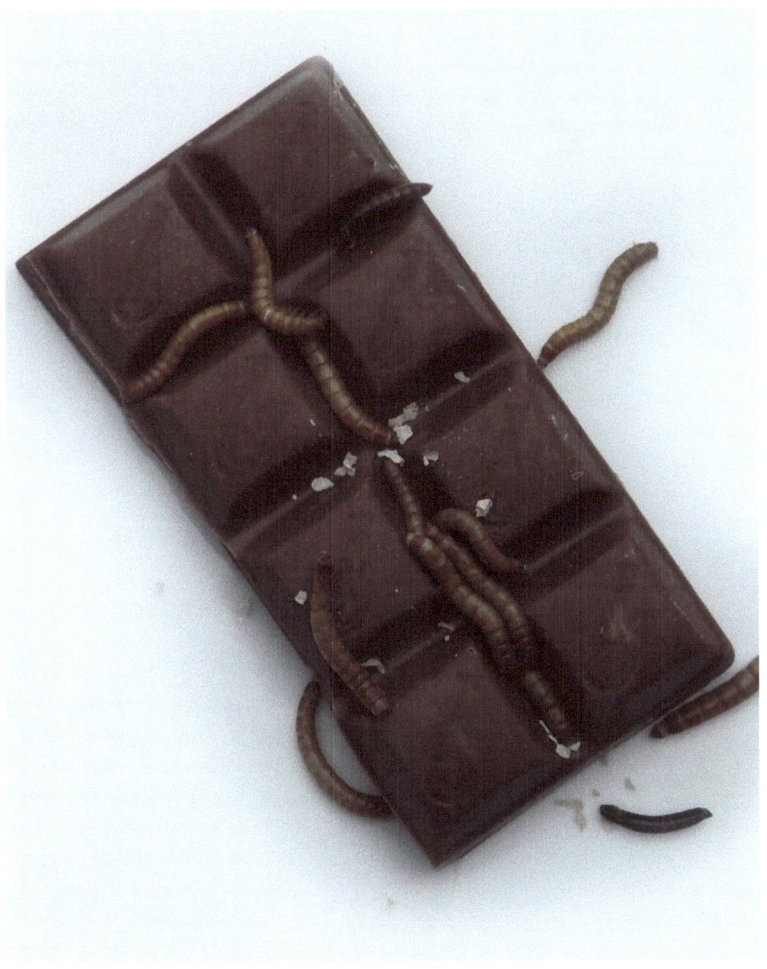

They wriggle. Blerg!
Ruined. Revolting!

CHERK!

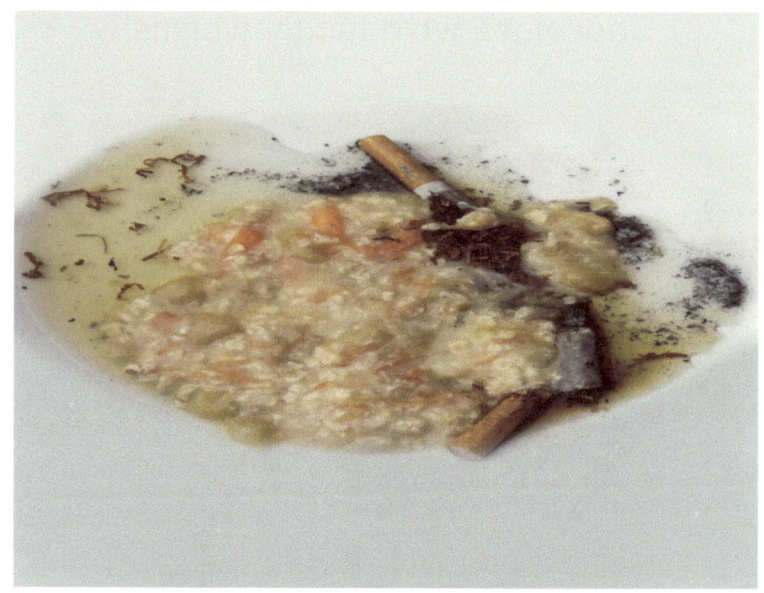

VOMIT - CHOCOLATE - SICK

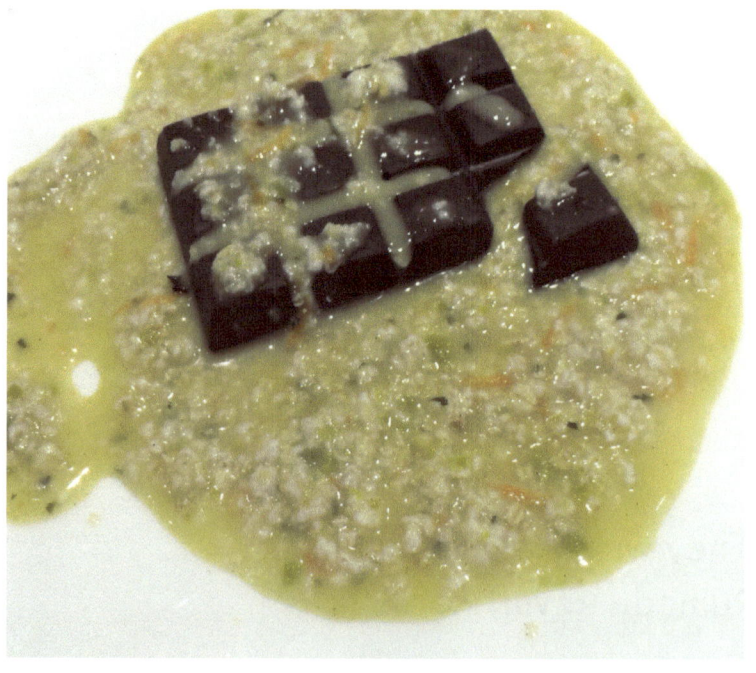

YUCK!

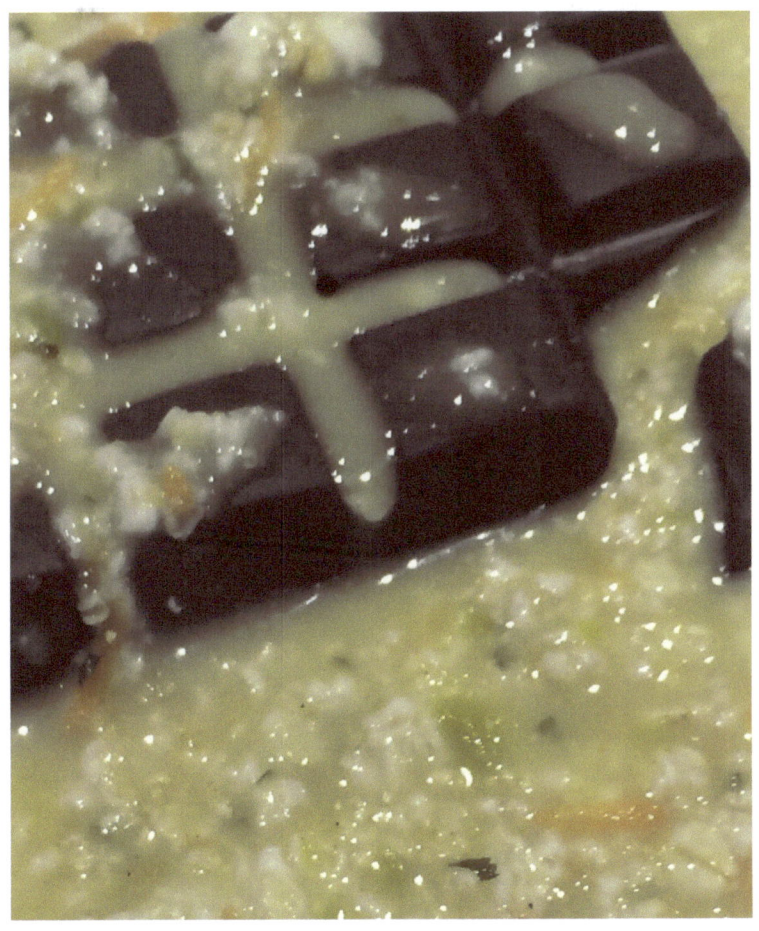

Be reminded of slimy vomit every time you think about eating chocolate. Smell it. URRGGH!

Yes. They are worms !

EEEEK!

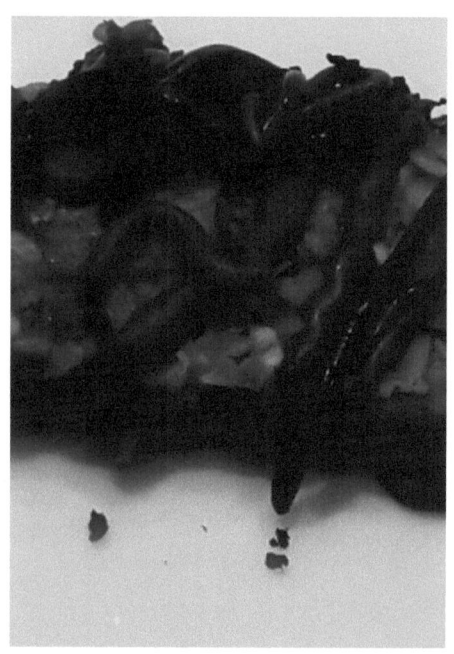

Brown, smooth and squirmy

Looks like chocolate. Aaaargh...

BLAH!
Chocolate with
        WORMS AND DIRT!

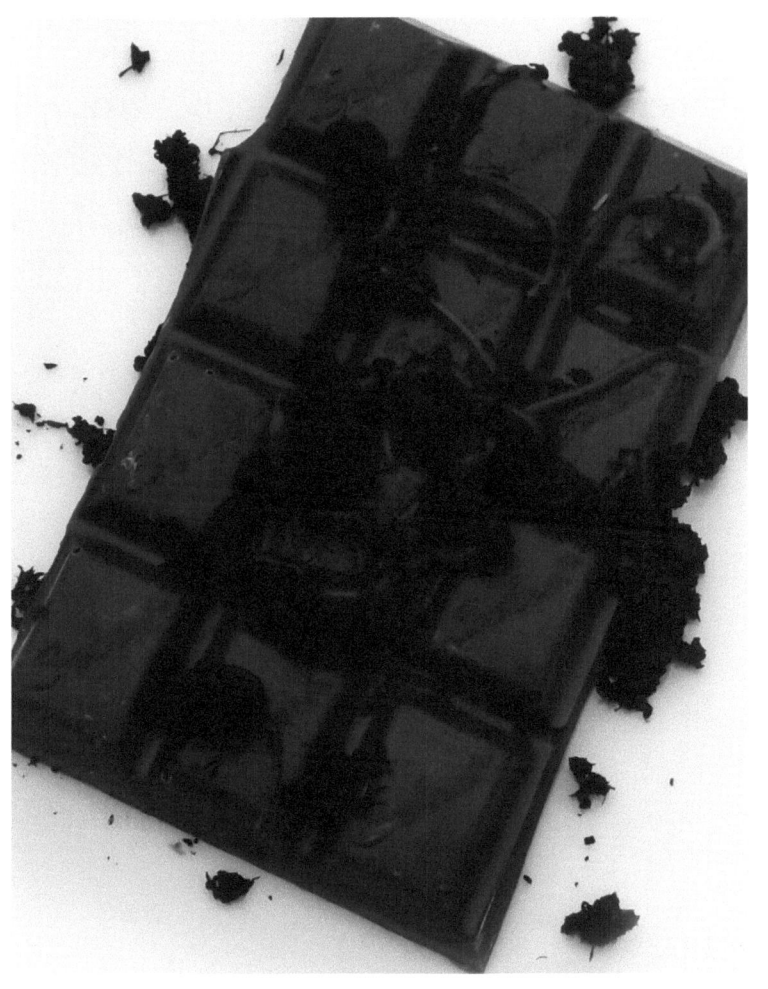

Slimy and dirty

YUCK!

Urrck! You know what that smells like! Putrid. Old Ash. Acrid vomit. Making you want to gag and retch. You know what it feels like. Slimy and sticky.

It reminds you of that chocolate you used to eat. Too much can be as bad for some people as cigarettes. The fat can clog their arteries and the sugar intake may lead to diabetes.

Diabetes can lead to premature death, loss of sight or toes, etc.

Be glad you have decided not to overindulge any more. You are freeing yourself from that old chocolate habit.

Revolting!

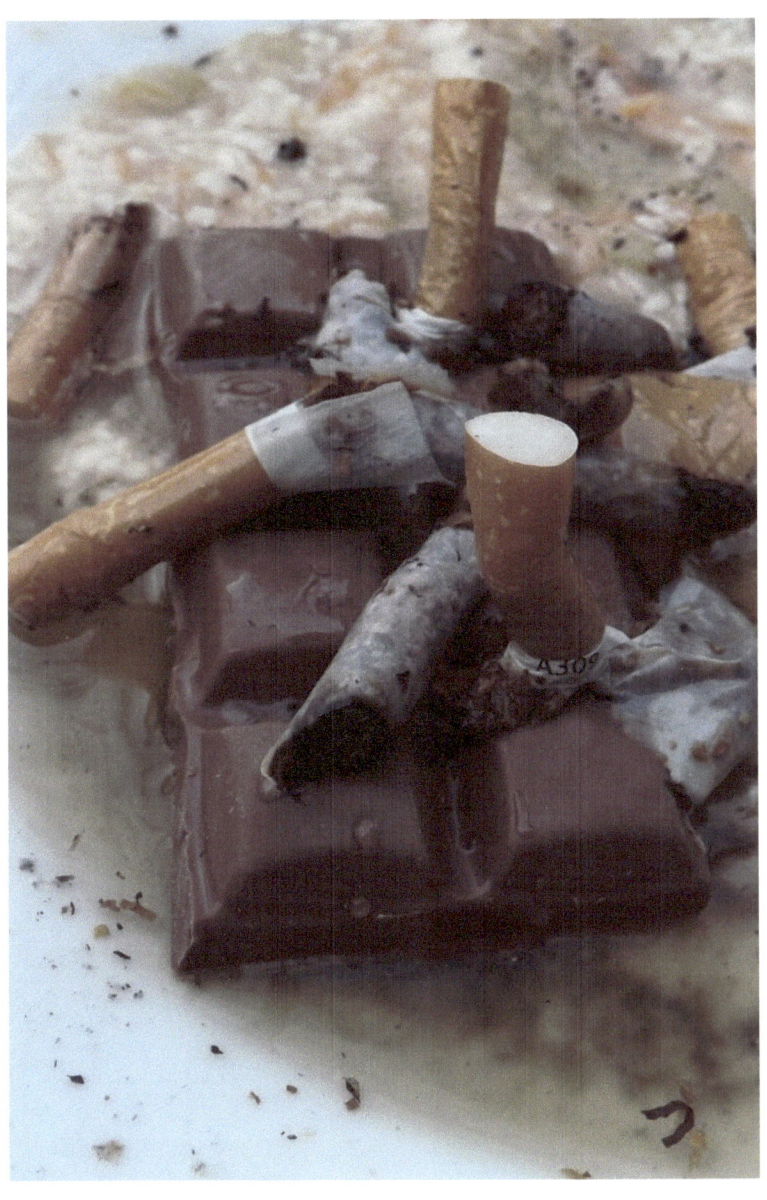

URRGH!

Mould!

Green, grey, white furry growth.

Smell it.

Feel it.

Associate that smell and feel with bringing chocolate to your mouth. That is one thing you no longer want to do ever again. Safely and comfortably avoid chocolate and mould.

URCK!

Mould !

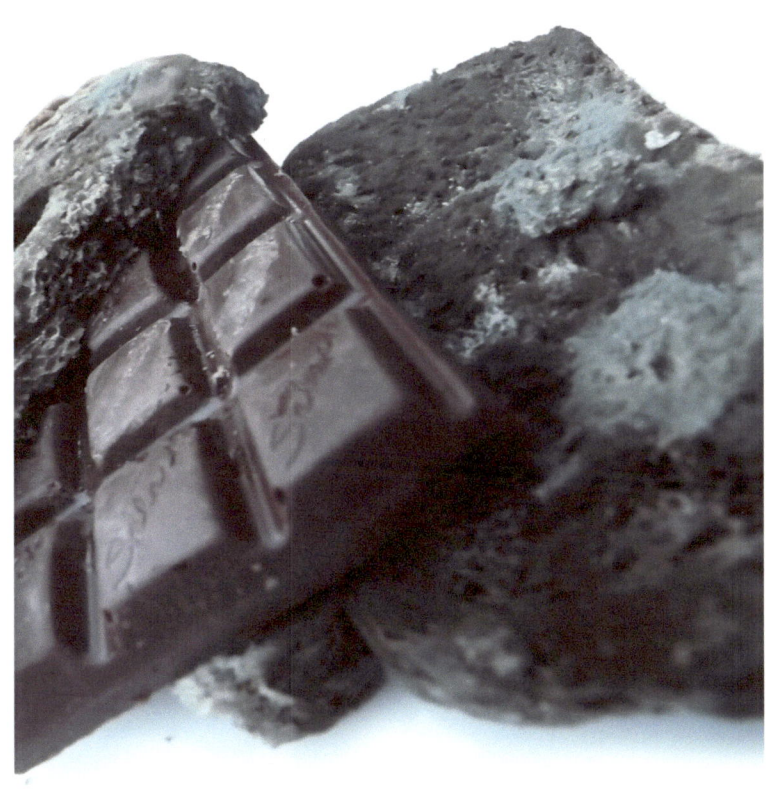

KEEP IT AWAY !

Mouldy chocolate sandwich?

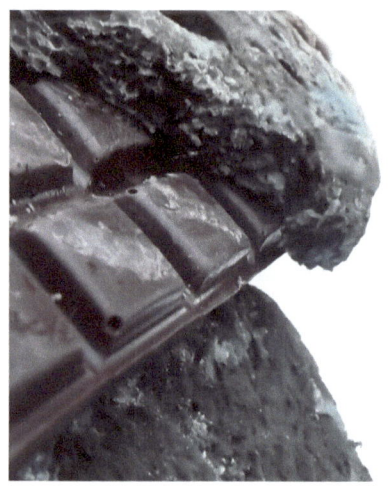

NO THANKS

Keep it out of your body

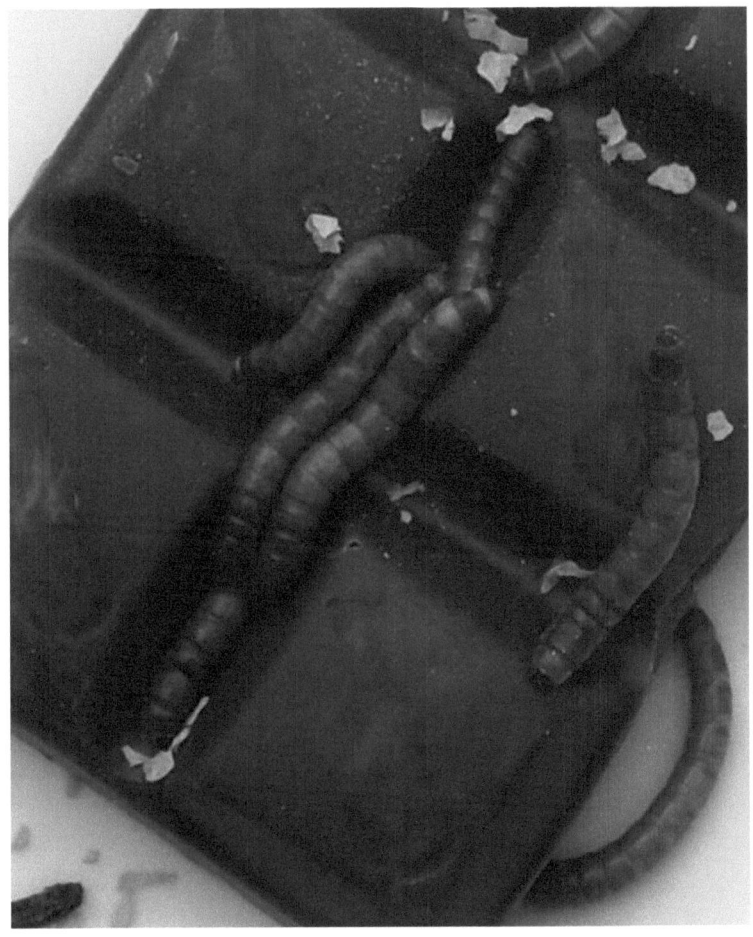

Chips on chocolate..
...or chips on shit?

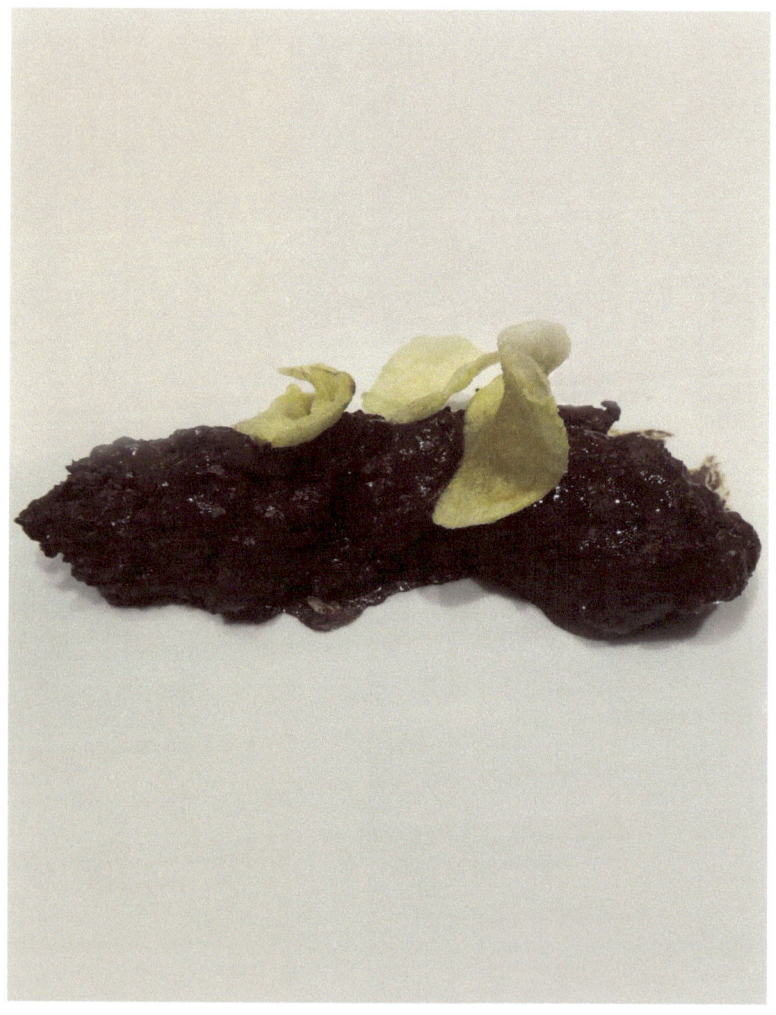

Chocolate addiction is shit.
It can look like it too.

Chocolate ? On the loo.

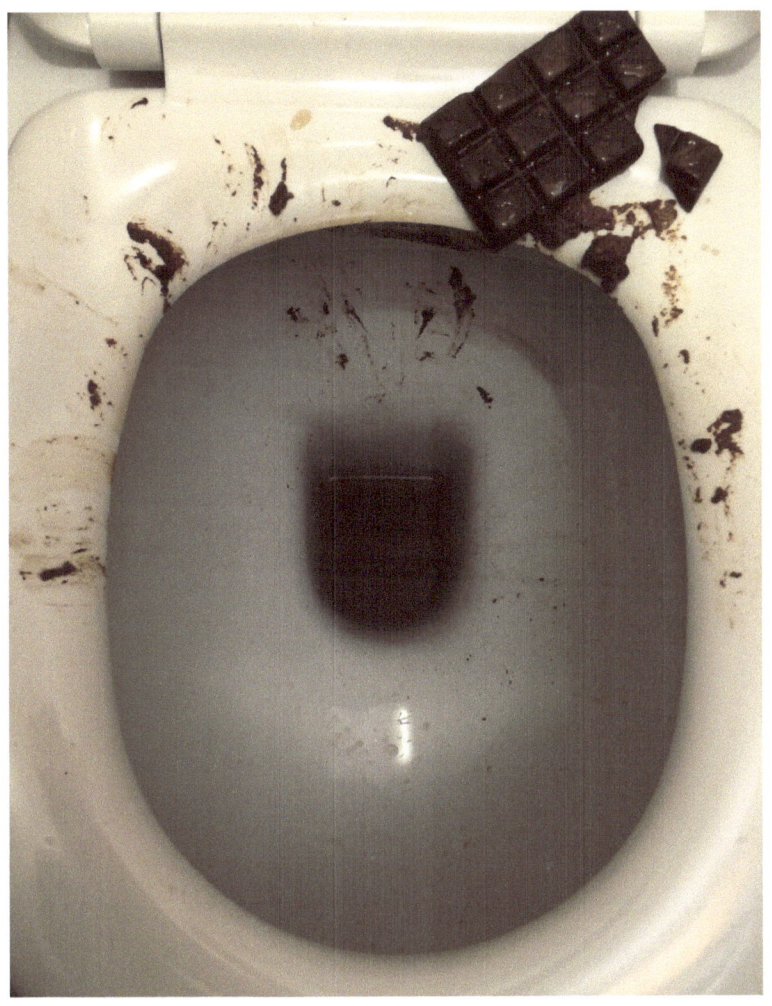

Before and after? Same, same.
Let it bypass your body.

POO

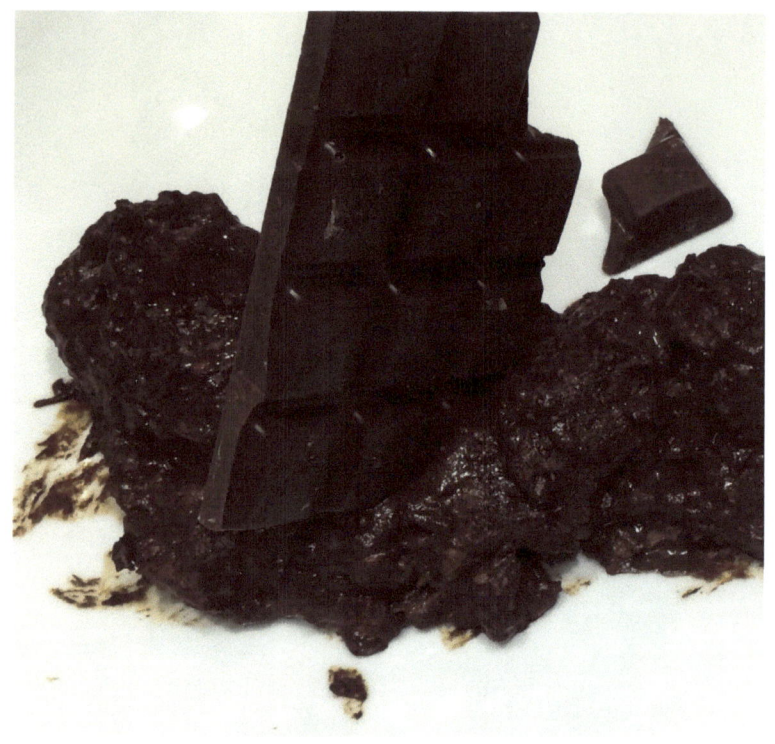

Would you put this on your hips from your lips?

Brown, slimy, gooey, fatty, greasy.

Chocolate can remind you of shit.

YURCK!

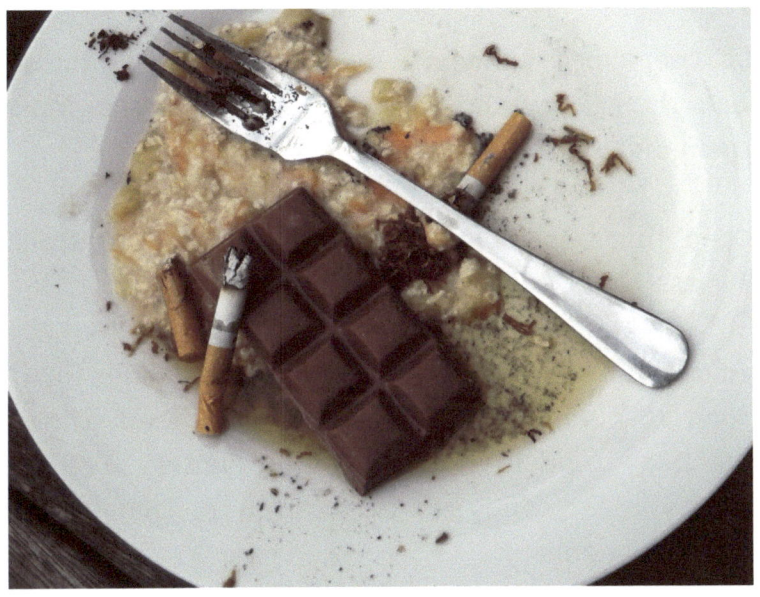

vomit, cigarette-butts, THROW IT OUT!

Perhaps you used to tamp down emotions with chocolate. You no longer need to do that. Just breathe deeply, drink water, relax, go for a walk.

You can let unwanted thoughts flow away. Thoughts are not facts unless you allow them to be.

If there are chocolate or sweets in the house, lock them away and forget where they are. Make them difficult to access.

Keep this book handy when you go to the store. Bypass the sweet section.

Value your body and only put good things in it. **Food is fuel.**. Only put in what you need. Ingest the best food with the best nutrients. You are what you eat. Only eat at mealtimes. Drink water between meals.

Love yourself. You are worth it.

STOP using yourself as a trash can

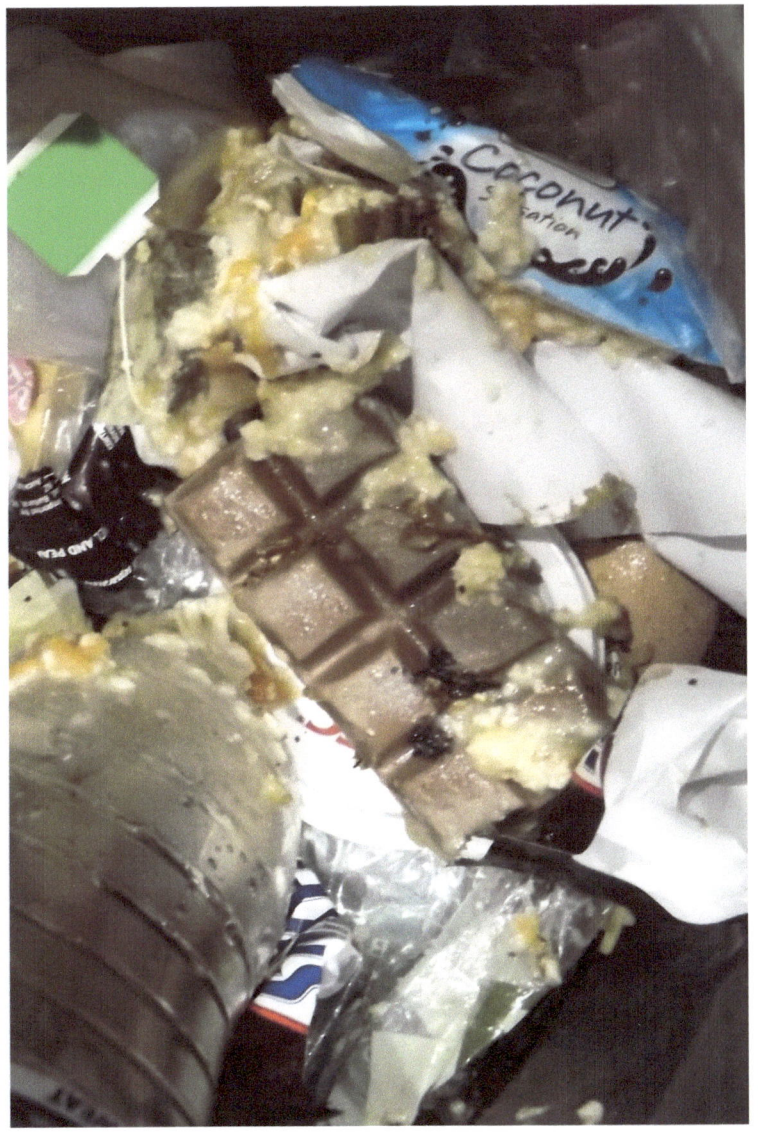

Chocolate is RUBBISH !

Instructions:

Are you ready to stop eating chocolate? If you really want to get rid of that old addiction you will need:

1. this book.

2. something that smells bad to YOU (e.g. rotten egg, surströmming - smelly Swedish tinned fish, rancid oil, off milk, diluted cleaning product, urinal balls, etc.).

3. (optional) something that tastes bad to YOU personally or e.g. smelly goats cheese, over-ripe bananas, Tabasco sauce, lemon, vinegar or vomit-flavoured jelly beans.

PROCEDURE

First:
Look at the picture of the chocolate on the first page. Note how much you would want to eat it (on a scale from 1 to 10).

Second:
Put the food you hate in your mouth and smell the substance that revolts you while looking at the rest of the pictures in the book. Spend at least a minute on each of the pictures you find revolting. Read. Imagine a better life free of that chocolate habit.

Third:
Look at the first picture again and notice how little you need it now in comparison (on a 1 to 10 scale).

Fourth:
Keep the book with you when you go shopping to remind yourself to connect chocolate with aversion.

Fifth:
Remember **PAUSE**

Punch the air 100 times, or go for a walk etc. to *pause* and avoid that revolting fatty, sugary sludge. You can get that good feeling from exercise instead.

Air can be breathed in deeply to relax you and fill you with energy and evaporate those old cravings.

Understand that you can drink **water** to wash away any future shadows of cravings. Many people are often only thirsty when they think they want to eat.

Select better, healthier food that will give you sustained energy: e.g. carrots, fresh fruit, a couple of nuts, or make a salad.

Ensure that chocolate and sweets are difficult to access: locked away or unavailable.

Welcome to a new life where you have control over those old addictions you used to have. You can remember to live without chocolate and sweets.

Disclaimer: no guarantees given for effectiveness. Pictures are planned to supplement the effect of an existing desire to stop eating chocolate, and help you to help yourself reduce mental cravings for it. Use common sense when selecting substances that smell or taste bad to supplement the therapy. Ensure they are safe, non-toxic and non-allergenic.

The End   =>   the first day of the rest of your life

www.ingramcontent.com/pod-product-compliance
Lightning Source LLC
Chambersburg PA
CBHW050929290526
45792CB00002B/941